MARRIAGE IS

FIFTY-FIFTY

AGY IRHEFO

MARRIAGE IS FIFTY-FIFTY

Agy Irhefo

© Copyright 2023 | Agy Irhefo

All scriptures, except otherwise stated, is gotten from the King James Version (KJV).

DEDICATION

This book is dedicated to every couple whose marriage needs a book like this home to build a beautiful marriage of their dream – full of bliss and blessings.

CONTENTS

PREFACE

Love indeed makes marriage but beyond that, it is important to also know that marriage is a spiritual institution. For this reason, the kind of love required to make a marriage work has a spiritual side too. It's a selfless and sacrificial love.

Love is a function of physical attraction and emotional connection, just like the fifty-fifty rule.

When you learn to see love this way, it is what makes you accept your spouse as who they truly are: beautiful but imperfect.

Love is expressed by people. When love grows, it culminates in marriage and it takes two people of opposite sex to make a marriage. People are a product of environmental influences. People are packs of diverging experiences.

As you commit to making your marriage work, sweet, and beautiful, you must carry this understanding that you're married to a person whose life has been shaped by environment and experiences that form his or her perspective and outlook that you're not privy to.

Have an open mind as you read this book. There are lessons you can glean from, and when you do, your home will be filled with bliss as you put them into practice.

CHAPTER ONE

MARRIAGE IS THE FULLNESS OF MANKIND

Man is a living soul. Man, when made, was fifty percent human (material body made from the dust of the ground) and fifty percent spirit (breath of the Almighty).

Man is a distinct being. He is totally and completely different from everything God created. When God was carrying out creation, He called everything to be and they became. He said "Light be" and there was light. The same process applied to the other creations. When it got to man's turn, God said "Let us MAKE man..." The man was not created, the man was made.

When God said, "Let us make man..." He was not referring to the man called Adam. Yes, God was not referring to a person. Note: God said "Let US..." God is a God of family. God understands the needs of species and kind. When He created creeping animals, beasts of the ground, and birds of the air, He created them after their kinds. When it got to man, the pattern didn't change.

Man in ancient Hebrew is ish and it refers to mankind. The Hebrew word Ish (man) is plural. So God said let US (our kind) make mankind. God was expressing an idea. In that idea of mankind, there was a male man and a female man but the male was made first.

After the first male man called Adam was made, and being a distinct being who was completely different from other creations, he was alone. Note that Adam was alone but not lonely. He was alone as he was the only one on the surface of the earth made after the order of his kind. Remember that other creatures God created were created after the order of their kind.

It was God who said, "It is not good for the man (Adam) to be alone." As we proceed, you will see why God said it is not good for man to be alone. Adam would need a company of his kind in the garden to not be alone. This is why the experiment that was carried out where the beast of the field and birds of the air were brought to Adam but his condition of aloneness wasn't cured. None was found suitable and complimentary.

What does this mean?

Adam was fifty percent God's vision. Do you now see why God said it is not good for Adam to be alone?

Let me break it further. Adam was half God's making of mankind. In essence, the mankind God referred to was not complete with only Adam on the Earth, and that was why

God said it was not good. When God created other creations, after looking at each, He said "It was good" but for Adam, it was not good.

The other half was required to be made so that it would be good. To complete the vision of "Let us make man...," the second fifty was made so that mankind can be expressed in its fullness.

Now that you already know that the second fifty percent was female man, how was this man made?

This time, instead of repeating the process through which Adam was made using the dust of the ground, God approached the process using a different method.

But why use a different method?

I will show you.

Think about the energy that produces electricity. If you have two positive charges, these two will not generate electricity. Even if you have ten, you still won't produce electricity without a negative charge. The energy that produces electricity is not complete in the absence of either of them. Note that for electricity to be produced, the presence of a negative charge is what completes the process of electricity generation, and vice versa.

In the same manner, for the man (mankind God referred to) to be made, there needed to be the making of a female man - Eve to complete and complement Adam.

CHAPTER TWO

THE FIFTY-FIFTY RULE

A scientist was asked, "Between a negative and a positive charge, which do you think is stronger?" He took some time off to carefully think and research before he gave his answer. This was what he had to say:

"No, we cannot tell that positive charge is stronger than negative charge or negative is stronger than positive charge or the charge of an electron is greater than the charge of a proton or vice versa."

The world's incomprehensiveness of this rule is why the world suffers gender discrimination. Today, there's an ongoing lopsided conversation about gender inequality brewing everywhere. These conversations are gradually becoming agitations that are setting up one gender against the other. Until people get it right, they will continue to chase shadows of equality of gender.

There's no basis for equality. Surprise?

Don't be yet.

I will show you why.

It is a vain effort to continue to insist that a woman is better than a man. In the same manner, it is a complete waste of energy to assert that a man is better than a woman. Unlike the positive and negative charge, we can tell that there's no basis for comparison between the male man and the female man. They are not equals, between them, there's no superior and there's no inferior.

I will further buttress why I told you that there's no basis for the comparison. Sit tight!

Let me give you a shocker. The global movement for gender equality is not the solution to gender discrimination. The solution to gender discrimination is simple. Yes, it is very simple. It is gender in-discrimination. It may not be a whole word in the English dictionary but it simply means the act of not indiscriminating against a gender. To put an end to discrimination against a certain gender is not the same as agitating for gender equality.

If you want the white skin to stop discriminating against the brown skin, does that mean the brown skin should become white, or like the white? no. It means let white be white and let brown be brown.

The female man was made because it was the only way to COMPLETELY solve the problem of man's aloneness. In Chapter One, I have shown to you what God meant when He said 'It is not good for Adam to be alone.'

There was something in the Bible that you need to know. "Be fruitful, and multiply; fill the Earth and subdue it; have dominion..." Who did God speak these words to?

THEM.

Who is them?

Man.

Recall that man is a plural word.

Truth is, if you don't look deeper, you'd assume that God was speaking only to Adam.

Where was Eve at the time when God spoke?

Think about it for a second.

I will ask for the second time. Where was Eve when God spoke saying "Be fruitful, and multiply; fill the Earth...?"

She was somewhere in the body of Adam.

You would see it in how the Bible rendered it. It said, "Then God blessed THEM..."

Now, you do understand that the fifty-fifty rule is not to set the Adams and the Eves against each other. Rather, the rule is to assert the distinctiveness of the Eves and the uniqueness of the Adams.

CHAPTER THREE

INSTITUTIONALIZATION OF MARRIAGE

It is typical of us to enter a house and expect that that house would be organized in a certain way so long as there's a woman in that house. Funny also is how unorganized we expect a house to be when there's no woman in that house. These are the expectations we enter a house with.

Think about it.

The truth however is not farfetched from how we think of these two sets of realities: an organized house because of the presence of a woman and an unorganized house because of the absence of a woman.

This was why God said 'It is not good for the man to be alone.' The man needs his second fifty to complete him.

So, God caused the man (Adam) to fall into a deep sleep. Then, He opened up Adam's body and took out a strong bone from the most fragile part of his body - the rib bone.

The rib bone doesn't look strong but it is strong enough to support the skeleton and protect the vital organs in the chest cavity, especially the heart. How strong can a bone be?

Have you ever wondered why God didn't use one of the bones in the toes of Adam? Or, maybe a bone in his hand?

While I want to leave you to ponder on these questions, I will proceed to show you something. We will return to the questions soon.

No matter how decent, focused, and disciplined a young man is, so long as he is still single, he is still perceived by society as "irresponsible." Society doesn't know how else to respond and relate to an eligible single who is not married. Society's response to his status is termed "irresponsible" as it is the only word that closely explains his incompleteness. Society's response is only an "unconscious effort" that supports God's verdict that IT IS NOT GOOD FOR A MAN THAT IS ELIGIBLE TO NOT BE COMPLETE.

In some places, they say the introduction of the woman into a man's life signifies the availability of the womb. Hence, the 'WO' that is added to 'MAN' (that is, adding a woman through the process of marriage to a man) is to make a womb available for the man. Therefore, the woman is an element of procreation. I don't disagree with that but marriage is not predicated on procreation. Making children is neither marriage nor the essence of marriage. Making children is a product of marriage.

Let me buttress it. The coming together of a man and a woman is not primarily to make children. Primarily, God wants a male man to function as a complete man. God wants a woman to function as a complete man. This is the mystery of one.

In marriage, a man will leave his father and mother and cleave to a woman he calls wife. These two people shall become ONE. In the scheme of God's agenda, these two people is MAN.

Genesis 2:24

This is also why marriage is fifty percent physical and fifty spiritual.

Now let's talk about the rib bone. God chose a rib that was close to the heart because of companionship. Companionship is the feeling of a sense of closeness that a person feels towards another. The man's heart must have this yearning feeling towards the woman.

When God brought to Adam the woman He had made for him, Adam exclaimed wow. He felt the connection from the first sight. So when he saw her, he said indeed, this is now the bone of my bones and the flesh of my flesh." Recall that the first experiment didn't get a match for Adam when the animals were brought to him. There was no connection. That was why he said 'This is NOW...'

Can you try to imagine how he responded? It must be a wow moment. It was the wow effect he must have exclaimed that made up why he said "She shall be called 'woman' for she was taken out of man' and formed for man.

CHAPTER FOUR

THE PURPOSE OF MARRIAGE

If you see me on the street or in the grocery store and ask me "Agy, what is the purpose of marriage?" My answer would be capsuled in three sentences:

1. It is a platform for companionship

2. It is a pledge to support a special person

3. It is a commitment to add value to a person.

Before I talk about all these three, let me ask you a question.

Why do you think young eligible bachelors and spinsters are losing interest in getting married?

Or, why do you think they delay the thought and decision to get married?

It is because those who went ahead of them were not properly schooled about marriage in their premarital days before they indulged in it. In essence, they have not seen good examples to model after.

A most recent research statistics (2023) shows that remarriage rates are higher among men than women. Buttressing this, it states that divorced men have 64% of remarriage while divorced women have 52% but here comes the shocker: 60% of remarriages end up in divorce. What this means is that 52% of divorced men and women who got married end up in divorce. Let me tell you the part of this statistics I find very interesting, it is that the rate of divorce in first-time marriages is less than that of remarried couples.

Shocking!

This points out that there's so much work to do. People need to be taught the purpose of marriage. That way, they would know what they are getting themselves involved in. So, let's talk about the purpose.

1. Platform for Companionship

It is about a company. Life is a journey, a very long one at that, and you must be careful about the person you want to be paired with in sailing through the journey. Marriage is about bringing two people who enjoy each other's company together. This aligns with the popular saying that 'two is a company and three is a crowd.' Nobody should take the place of your spouse, not even your children. This is because your spouse is the person who has a permanent place by your side and will remain at your side till the end even after every other person leaves. Your children will eventually leave. Friends will leave. It does not mean that they are bad people. It is how is programmed.

Marriage presents us with the opportunity to have a partner - someone you can call "your own." We all have a longing for that, the longing to have someone to call 'mine.' And usually, that is a person you have unhindered access to. When all is said and done, you will discover that sex in marriage is subject to a functional age but companionship is a lifetime affair.

2. Pledge Support for a Person

Perfection is an illusion. There's no perfect partner in a marriage. Human beings have certain weaknesses.

Everybody desires to have someone who identifies and understands their weakness and provide support for them in that area. This is the reason why it is fundamentally important for everyone who desires to get married to build value in themselves first. As a woman, you would need to provide financial counsel to your husband. A times, you would be required to provide office administrative counsel too.

The nature of support you would be required to provide for your partner is varied. It can be emotional, financial, etc.

3. Commitment to Add Value

The wise King Solomon said in Ecclesiastes "Two are better than one; because they have a good reward for their labor. For if they fall, the one will lift his fellow." Marriage is a full-time work. It is a commitment to work tirelessly to make your spouse better, and you work daily. You work round the clock.

Yes, we have asserted that marriage is work and the purpose of this work is primarily designed to better your spouse. This, in essence, means to add value to your spouse. So, how do you add value to your spouse?

Be interested and be involved in their daily activities. Try to inquire about what they are involved in and make input.

Have a desire to inquire what they are thinking and show concern.

Hold them accountable for the goals they set. Provide support and advice to them and ensure that they stay true to their goals until they achieve them.

Help them wind down after every hectic day or stressful activity. Tell a story, or give a massage, or give a pleasurable sex. We will talk about sex and intimacy in the next chapter.

Everything I have said about the purpose of marriage is from a human standpoint. If you put the purpose of marriage in a divine perspective, you will discover that it is completely different. Firstly, marriage is between two adults and these adults must be of opposite genders. The Bible says that it is because of marriage that a man will leave his father and mother, that man has to be an adult who is old enough as well as responsible enough, to be joined to a woman. The decision about gender is not a man's to make. From the beginning, God decided on it. Hence, male and female created He them.

There is a reason a boy is born as a boy. There is a reason why a girl is born as a girl. You probably want to ask me "What is the reason?" My answer will be "I didn't create anyone." The One who creates knows why.

CHAPTER FIVE

SEXUAL INTIMACY

In the intimate life of a couple, it is important to assert that there are never more than two parties in this place. It is an affair between two people. This is why porn is so dangerous. It is a deadly stranger. When you invite or allow a stranger into your intimate space, you violate the law that states that 'there are never more than two parties.' Yes, there's no room for anyone else.

Let me tell you this. Whenever you allow pornography into your intimate space, you're inviting a third party. Because of the law of intimacy, there will be an insistence that ONLY TWO PEOPLE SHOULD BE INVOLVED IN THIS SPACE. Hence, its implication will create a circumstance that will lead to the eviction of one party.

Who's it going to be?

The porn?

The woman?

Or the man?

You have to decide.

When marriage happens, intimacy must be established between the two of them ONLY. Without intimacy, their relationship in that marriage is simply mechanical. Sex is not intimacy, even though sex is required for intimacy to become complete in some cases. This must be clearly stated. Sex is good. Sex is needed. But, intimacy is better.

Intimacy is a place established between a husband and a wife. This place, no one else is allowed because it is the heart of the home and it also holds the very covenant upon which the marriage is enacted.

A lot of couples find it difficult to function as they should in this place of intimacy. Because of various distractions, a lot of couples reduce what should be intimacy into sex. Distractions like:

Kids: When the union starts making babies, intimacy begins to dwindle, and usually because of this, the couple reduces their intimate experience to sex. With the coming of kids, the couple's attention begins to focus on their children and this creates a lacuna.

Boredom: After a while of having sex with your spouse, the experience becomes boring.

Emotional disconnectedness: More than the "distractions" the kids create, when couples begin to settle into the monotony of life (work) and the financial pressure to keep the home together, the passion between the couple begins to evaporate. At this stage, the majority of the conversation between the couple is about bills.

Oftentimes, as they make an effort to rekindle their intimate affair, they "invite a stranger." Usually, they condescend to using porn. Don't forget. Porn is a not-go-to place.

Intimate Sex

Marriages fail and one of the reasons why it fails is sex. However, it is important to clarify this. Most times, it is not the absence of sex. Rather, it is the absence of intimacy. Intimacy is about an internal connection while sex is about a physically pleasurable activity. Even though sex happens in the physical, it has invisible components, and it is these invisible components that qualify it to be termed as intimacy. Let me demonstrate this.

A person who wants to eat is different from the person who needs to eat. The former is concerned about the food (health benefits, dietary plan, and nutritional components), the experience to get from the process of eating the food, and the outcome as well. The latter who needs to eat simply wants to cure hunger. Even though the physical activity the former and latter might be engaged in might be similar, there's still a difference.

That difference is what you would liken to the difference between intimacy and sex.

It is important you know that intimacy is about building emotional, mental, trust, and honorable affairs between a husband and his wife. In other words, it means sex can happen in the absence of intimacy but intimacy, most times, is sex and more.

For you and your spouse, you must ensure that your sexual relationship and experience is intimate all the time. The main thing to catch here is simple. It is the fact that there is a process to this thing happening. A lot of times, spouses don't pay attention to the process that creates intimacy, rather they focus on satisfying their sexual needs. Sex is selfish. Intimacy is different. My suggestion to you is to begin with a foot rub. Then, you will discover that it is about making your partner feel good in every way you can. A Foot rub is just one random example, you can think about other ways too, like back rubs and massages. Through these simple things, you communicate tender love and care to your spouse and this is so important.

Am I saying couples cannot have sex? I mean just sex, like a quickie? Of course, they can. It's fun and that's it. A quickie is fun and it is a bit of an adventure. Nothing more. This is something you can liken to sushi. Couples don't do sushi every time. Yes, couples don't have quickies often.

CHAPTER SIX

COMMUNICATION IN MARRIAGE

Couples need to learn how to talk about their home and about what is working and what is not working between them. The only time most couples get to talk is when there's a disagreement or misunderstanding. It becomes the avenue they take to speak up but it doesn't always help because, for some people, they bottle up a lot of things in their chest for a long time. When a misunderstanding finally presents them with the opportunity to pour out, they don't hold back. Sometimes, it leaves their partner in awe because they never knew their spouse had so much heaped in their minds all along.

Normally, it should be expected that when a partner pours out so much at once, addressing all of them and making necessary adjustments can become overwhelming.

You should learn to talk to your partner every time. If you're not satisfied with the way he or she is handling something, find the best way to bring it up. Don't wait until things go wrong or when you have a misunderstanding.

Sometimes, some partners don't like to talk. They simply react. When you try to ask them why they are putting up a face or giving an attitude, they give short responses. Usually they say "Nothing." If your partner is like that, you have a responsibility to help them understand that it is not healthy for your marriage. Don't talk about it when they are in that mood. Wait until you're both having a great moment together to bring it up and let them know how their silence hurts you. As you do this, affirm your commitment to learn and to make amends so that your marriage can work. Let them know you cannot learn and make amends where necessary if areas of your imperfections or inadequacies are not pointed out clearly to you. Help them to see how teachable you are willing to be.

Always learn to take stocks. Once in a while, pause and ask your spouse "What am I not doing right?"

Your spouse will point those things to you in the best possible way he or she can without making you feel bad or less of yourself.

Assuming you ask your spouse "What am I not doing right?" during a heated argument, trust me, you won't have the strength to carry the answer you will get.

It's the same question. But the answers will be different. The difference is in the timing.

As a man, when you communicate with your spouse, do it as you would with anyone on your sideline. It doesn't matter whether you're 15 years older in age, if she's your wife, she's your sideline. The moment she became your wife, she joined the team of people in your league. She is your friend. You cannot talk to her the way you would a protege or mentee. You cannot talk to her the way you would a subordinate. She's your wife. By this, she is a co-you. You cannot be uptight and rigid with your wife. You would need her to help you see things from the perspective you cannot. You would need her counsel to make decisions.

As a woman, you must learn to deal with your husband using a dual approach because he is both your sideline and upline. As your sideline, you will relate with him as your friendship. As your upline, you will relate with him with reverence because he is your head - your leader and your covering. In fact, he is your first pastor.

This is such a difficult thing to do without the help of the Holy Spirit.

Think about it.

How do you see your husband as your lord whom you owe a responsibility to serve, and also see him as a friend whom you talk and play with, and sometimes argue with?

It is such an enormous responsibility, yet so delicate.

Fights: Disagreement and Misunderstandings

When couples fight, it is a strategy of the devil to cause division between them. They will be so close but yet so distant from each other. Why do you think it is common to find couples raising their voices when they quarrel? So close but yet too distant. An attack on marriage is not an attack on the individuals in the marriage, it is an attack on their power. Recall that we have established that couples generate power from the place of their unity. When couples quarrel and fight, it sets their hearts far apart from each other. When they are connected in unity, they can communicate without really talking. When they talk, they do so subtly with smooth, quiet, and soothing voices.

But how does a fight begin among couples?

Argument.

An argument begins with two things: disagreement and misunderstanding.

Disagreement ensues when one partner holds a contrary opinion or belief about a thing, an idea, a person, or even a place. In expressing your disagreement, you can communicate it without putting it forward as an attack or even make your partner perceive your point as an attack.

Think about this: God is the only one in His class. No human can match up to God. Yet, God allows Himself to come to the table and reason with humans. He said "Come, let us reason together..." In essence, if you don't agree with some things, come, let us reason about it together. If you don't like something, come, let us reason about it together. This is how He reasoned with Job. In reasoning together, one party may cross the limit, it is the other party's responsibility to bring to order his or her partner.

This is the reason why the Bible said, even when we attempt to correct a person, let's do it in love.

Misunderstanding comes from miscommunication. How do you speak to your spouse? Your spouse is not your boss, you don't shiver and quake when talking to them. Your spouse is not your subordinate. You don't speak to your spouse like you speak to your subordinate. Your spouse is half you. You must speak to your spouse with courtesy, just as you would want to be spoken to.

Season Your Words

Statistics show that over 80% of times when a couple sits before a counselor, the man complains about one thing: "She doesn't respect me." What this also means is that the woman stops perceiving and receiving the man as the head - her head, because the man has allowed the enemy to creep in.

Remember, every time the enemy comes around a home, he looks for an opportunity to seize the position of the man. Every opportunity he gets, he undermines the position of the man in the eyes of the woman. Consequently, the man feels disrespected. When the man feels disrespected, he disconnects himself from the spouse and that creates an avenue for the enemy. Usually, this condition degenerates into a quarrel.

The longer the quarrel lasts between the man and his wife, the longer the devil stays in charge; and the deeper the quarrel, the stronger influence and control the devil wields. The bitter the environment you create using hurtful words on each, the better that environment becomes for the devil to thrive.

This is why couples must learn not to use negative or hurtful words on their partners, no matter what. It is generally believed that women talk more than men. A study conducted by the School of Public Health (Harvard T. H.

Chan) shows that "context is the key to whether or not it is actually true." According to Sylvia Smith, women "tend to talk more - more often, at greater length and about more personal topics." Men, on the other hand, talk far more than women in formal settings like public speaking or business-focused contexts and meetings. From this, you know that in the home, the woman talks more. This is why the Bible in Proverbs 14:1 speaks about wise women as those who build their houses. It went on to say that the foolish pulls down her house with her own hands (thoughts, words, and actions).

But in Proverbs 14:3, the Bible went on to show one character of the foolish. It says "A fool's mouth lashes out with pride, but the lips of the wise protect them." Does this mean that one of the important ways a woman pulls down her home is her mouth? Think about it for a moment. A man feels respected and receives submission from his wife, first, in the way the woman talks to him. How she acts is second because it is the expression of what she says. It begins with how she talks.

Wisdom

In Proverbs 14:8, the Bible says "Stay away from a fool, for you will not find knowledge on their lips." I will ask you again, could it be that the Bible is instructing that it is a safe thing to do to stay away from women who do not use their lips wisely? Here's what I find very interesting: The Bible also identified them by their character: there's no knowledge found on their lips.

When a wise woman has her lips filled with knowledge, you will find her words gracious, soothing, and seasoned with salt. The Bible said in Proverbs 16:24 that "Gracious words are like a honeycomb, sweetness to the soul and health to the body." Your marriage becomes sweet and stays so when it's filled with gracious words. That's how to build your home and keep your marriage healthy.

A woman may not have ill intentions for her marriage but may be pulling down her home with her words. It is possible that her intentions are great and the things she does (including sacrifices she makes) for her marriage may be undermined by her lips. This is just how powerful words can be.

Words have creative power. It can create (build-up) or destroy (tear down) her house. The atmosphere in the home is largely a product of the nature of the words the couple uses in their words.

An example of the power in the tongue is what the Bible rendered saying that soothing words can turn away anger. The Bible rendered an example in Proverbs 15:1 saying that kind words turn away anger. In the same manner, harsh words stir up anger.

As a couple, the words you use on each other will come to manifest by affecting you both, it is self-deception to say "I don't care." You care. You simply say you don't care as a means to license you to speak unguarded words but you do care. That's why you're still there. You're still in the house with your spouse. You're still in the marriage with your spouse. When you utter hurtful words because you say to yourself that you don't care, you are hurting yourself too. When your partner is hurt, you're hurt too. Your partner cannot hurt alone. Because you're a couple, a part of you is already given to him or her and vice versa. It doesn't matter how you feel in the moment, you care. In the long run, you will realize you care, no matter what.

You host so much power when you cherish one another. You wield so much control when you love one another.

Responsibility to Self

It is also important that you know that your life was first independent before it became interdependent in marriage, and yet still, there's a level of independence that exists in interdependence. Your spouse will not always make you feel happy. You owe yourself a responsibility to build a positive mindset about yourself and it must come from what God says about you. When you're created, God said you're good the way you are created. If God said you're good and complete, it means you are. You should be able to build a perception of yourself based on God's word so much so that some words won't make you doubt because of words spoken to you. You have to learn to feel good about yourself. You have to learn to make yourself feel good by yourself. You have a responsibility to stay on watch and guard your joy.

The world is filled with so much negativity. People are quick to speak harshly. They are quick to speak hurtful words. Why are they slow to speak soothing and good words? You owe yourself that responsibility to speak reaffirming and empowering words to you. Beautiful words are not given to any particular gender. Both men and women enjoy beautiful words being spoken to them. Therefore, it means both the man and woman must learn to speak beautiful words to one another.

CHAPTER SEVEN

MARATHON OF COMMITMENT

It hurts the devil when your marriage is sweet. In the same way, the devil is happy when your marriage is hurting. But the good news is that it is within your power to disarm the devil. Just commit to making your marriage work. Your commitment is very important.

Commitment is not required only when your marriage is sailing well. Commitment is required every time. Through the thick and the thin, you must be committed to a single goal: make it work.

When couples use hurtful words against each other, the devil collects these words and uses them against them. Every hurtful word you use tears down your home. Words are very powerful. It can build and it can tear down.

In a home, where responsibility lies in the head. The man is not the head of the home because of his biceps. The head of the house is a position of leadership and leaders are identified by responsibility.

In every home, someone must be in a position of responsibility and that person is the go-to person when answers are sought. Whatever shape a home takes, it is the head of the house that gets to be asked because, as the head, he will be answerable.

There's no neutral ground. I mean, there's no home without a head. If the man is not assuming his position and taking his place as the head, someone will. There's usually one person who desires that the man does not live up to expectations as the head, it is the devil. Since there's no neutral home, whatever is the reason why the man abandons his position as the head, the devil will jump in and take over. This is the primary reason why the devil creates division in the home by causing misunderstanding and disagreement that leads to quarrels.

CHAPTER EIGHT

MINISTRY OF FORGIVENESS

Forgiveness is something we are taught by demonstration. God created man, in the beginning, and man sinned against the God that created him. God forgave man in a way He demonstrated the depth and gravity of what was required for such forgiveness. It was to the end that we should learn. We are not perfect. As spouses, learning forgiveness is a MUST because you can never get a married partner anywhere. A perfect partner doesn't exist.

Your partner will err. You will also err. Knowing that we are who we are because of God's ministry of forgiveness called mercy, you must learn to be empathetic and merciful to your spouse.

Forgiveness is not an act, it is a state of being. You must perpetually the in that state. This is why some people say things like "having the spirit of forgiveness" to refer to it as a spirit people embody. This is important because your spouse will not err once. In the Bible, a Christian is admonished to forgive ONE person seventy- seven times. Can you pause and think about this for a moment? You are required to forgive ONE person seventy-seven times, how about the next person, and the next, and the next? You would need to perpetually be forgiving to do that. This is why I said it is a state of being, not an act.

Interestingly, you find peace within yourself only when you forgive. How can you not forgive when you want to find peace within yourself? Every successful marriage is wrapped around the spouse's ability to express forgiveness towards themselves. Sometimes, forgiveness looks hard. What it looks like is not important. What is important is that it is possible. When you forgive, you will stop being bitter, your spirit will feel lightened and you will have wisdom and direction for the next level. When you harbor unforgiveness, you will be blind and you will feel like you're carrying weight. You cannot feel the inner peace you deserve. Forgiveness is a MUST.

You're much more powerful than you think, you can do great things but unforgiveness is strong enough to stop you if you allow it. Most times, when you feel like not forgiving your spouse, it is the devil's plot and trap to steal your power. The devil knows how much power is domiciled in you and how much of this power you can generate in union with your spouse. His attack strategy is to render you powerless first then he steals your peace. The more you refuse to forgive, he moves further to steal your joy by overloading you with unnecessary burdens and blinds you from making the right decisions because you feel disconnected from your wells of wisdom.

Do you wonder why?

Forgiveness is not a sign of weakness. It is a symbol and demonstration of strength.

CHAPTER NINE

POWER OF APPRECIATION

Appreciation is powerful. It brings an increase. Unlike what most people think, appreciation is not gratitude. Gratitude is the state of being thankful, and don't get me wrong, being thankful is very important. You must cultivate a culture and an attitude of always being grateful and saying thank you to your spouse for the little things and the big things. When you are grateful and you express your gratitude over something your spouse does for you, it obligates your spouse to do it again and even outdo himself or herself.

Appreciation is quite different. According to Rick Warren, gratitude is an attitude but appreciation is a spirit. Appreciation breeds an environment for increase. It is not just a response to what your spouse is, it is about who your spouse is and how you value the position they occupy. Do you know what appreciation does to your partner? It makes them feel wanted. It makes them feel noticed. It makes them feel desired. It makes them special and important. Appreciation is one of the things that ensures everything grows in your home. This is because it is one thing that wants to make any person bring his or her A-game to spice up their union. Think about it. Won't you give your best to a person that makes you feel special? Won't you do your best in a union where you are valued? This is why appreciation is so important. It helps with the emotional well-being of any couple. It spices the sex life of every couple because the partners both feel noticed, wanted, and desired as well.

In a marriage, it is not only financial stability that guarantees security. It takes more than money. In fact, it requires more than finance and faithfulness to one partner. Appreciation makes a partner feel good about the marriage union they are in and about the person they are in the union with. This is the most important factor that gives a partner the most feeling of security in marriage.

When you become intentional about appreciating your partner, your partner gets the most assurance that you are conscious about him or her.

This is why it is necessary to look at your partner in the eye and say to them things like:

I thank God for you.

I thank God for the kind of person you are.

I thank God for bringing us together.

I thank God for bringing you into my life.

My life is better and sweet because you're in my life.

Appreciation helps you to focus on the strength of your partner. When you shower appreciation, you help your partner to see the good in them and to believe more in themselves.

Why do you think school uses after-school routines as punishment for children in school? It is because they know how children long for home after school hours. To the child, there's no place like home. The child longs to run home to mummy. Usually, it's not about the mummy, it's about the environment the mummy creates for that child. That's what appreciation does to the home of couples.

Appreciation is how you detoxify your home environment because your partner always wants to come home running to you. There's no other place he or she gets that feeling except with you or around you. Appreciation has a greater effect on men than it does on women. A compliment works well on the woman.

When you have learned to appreciate your partner as you ought to, it does one thing. It brings your partner to the realization that no one cares for them as you do, and no one would ever will.

This feeling of assurance is ecstatic.

CHAPTER TEN

FORCE OF COMPLIMENTS

You don't wait for the big things. You don't wait for outstanding things. You don't wait for the ravishing looks or classy dress or attire. Make compliment a culture in your marriage.

Compliments are really more than kind words. Science has shown that when we receive honest compliments from our loved ones, our brains release a chemical called dopamine. Dopamine is a pleasure hormone. It is a chemical that makes humans feel good. This feeling is placed in the same category as the feeling people get when they reach orgasm during sex. Researchers believe that giving compliments activates the striatum in them. The striatum is one of the reward areas in the brain.

A compliment has a mood-lifting effect. Listen, the art of giving simple but honest compliments can make a huge difference in your marriage.

In an article published in marriage.com, Sylvia Smith shares different ways a lack of compliments can ruin marriages. Are you surprised? Don't be. A lack of compliments ruins marriages.

Like a man wants appreciation, women want compliments more than men.

Your hair smells nice.

Your skin is soft and sweet.

Your legs are beautiful in those skirts.

These short and simple words give the woman the guarantee that you're thoughtful of her and she's also desirable to you.

There's a connection between appreciation and compliments. The sad truth is that one triggers the other in a forward and backward linkage. If the man stops giving compliments to the woman, she's likely going to cease appreciating him and vice versa.

One of the reasons why couples stop giving compliments or appreciation to their partners is when they start to become overly critical of their partner. No one is perfect. There are better ways to communicate their inadequacies. Another reason is when they start to become busy. Never become too busy to notice your partner and make them feel valued, no matter what. In the long run, all the busyness will be useless if you lose your partner whom you're busy with. That's my counsel.

CHAPTER ELEVEN

MAGIC OF GRATITUDE

Some women have nagged their husbands out of the house. The man just left and didn't come home because of ingratitude and ceaseless nags.

The Bible said in Proverbs 21:9, it is better to live on the corner of the roof than to share a house with a nagging wife.

This is not surprising at all.

Some men spend hours out with the boys after work because coming home to their wife who nags is a nightmare they can't bear to face long before bedtime. For some men, it is a nightmare they can't bear to face without being intoxicated with alcohol.

This is sad.

Listen, you don't have to wait for your husband to buy you that SUV or sports car before you say thank you.

For the candy he buys you, tell him "Thank you."

When he takes out and empty the bin, tell him "Thank you."

For the groceries he buys or the money he provides for the groceries, you should express gratitude.

When he pays for the cable, internet, or electricity bills, say to him "Thank you."

When the children's school fees are paid, tell him "Thank you." Teach the children to do the same when their school fees are being paid or when daddy pays for the cable.

You must also teach them to say thank you when they are taken out for ice cream or when Daddy buys them toys.

Gratitude must be made a culture in your home if you want to enjoy your marriage.

We have established that the presence of the woman brings organization into the man's life. It is quintessential for the man to always learn to express gratitude to the woman for making his life organized. A man needs to learn to always express gratitude to his wife for always keeping his home habitable and clean. It is not proper for a husband to assume it is her default responsibility. It is not proper to assume that there's nothing special in a woman's making of the meal and keeping of the house. It takes effort to keep a house and make the meals. Say thank you to her ALWAYS.

When she fails to keep the house like she always does, it is improper to confront her with questions like "What have you been doing all day?" "Why is the house so dirty?"

Don't do that.

When you do that, it makes you a nagging husband, too.

What should you do instead?

Help her. Clean the house. Do it in her stead without grumbling. Secondly, thank her for all the times she has kept the home clean. Then, you can attempt to find out why she didn't keep the house like she always does.

CHAPTER TWELVE

THE *US*-MINDSET

In marriage, one thing you must learn to always do is to always put your partner in perspective.

Whatever you're doing, do not make it a me-thing. You need to know that in marriage, you're one with your partner. Therefore, you must ensure always that everything is in the interest of you both.

If possible, as much as you can always put your partner first before you. Your union becomes stronger and better when you're selfless when you put your partner first. It is important that in your home, create a culture of 'pleasing my partner first.'

Inculcate in yourself the ability to please your partner a priority.

Learn to always use the word US as you converse with your spouse. It is perspectives that make the marriage experience beautiful. It is so important that every time a woman wants to be heard, she should do it suggestively. Any time a woman goes out of her place to assert her opinion or perspective, two things are likely going to happen with the man:

1. A revolt

2. Irrationality

The man is a rational being. The man is slow to reach conclusions. In fact, a man takes his time to think something through before reaching a decision. This process is usually quite slow compared to the time a woman takes to think and reach a decision.

When he comes under pressure because of his wife's assertiveness, or when his desire to please his wife allows him to give in to his wife's assertiveness, he's likely going to make some irrational decisions that may haunt him.

As you grow in learning how to do this, ensure that you avoid opening another gap for the enemy. Avoid comparison because it will always create a rift and set you apart from your spouse.

One of the greatest undoings of marriage is comparison. Your marriage is different not because it was joined by a special pastor who has a unique anointing or because it was joined in the presence of special people in the audience to witness.

Your marriage is different and unique because you are unique and different. Your partner too. On the surface of the Earth, there's no one like you or your partner. Because of this, no marriage CAN ever be like yours.

Why compare your marriage with other's?

Why compare your partner with someone else's?

It is foolish. It is not an attitude that binds you and your spouse together.

When a man suddenly wants his wife to start dressing in a certain way, there's a high possibility that he saw someone's wife dressing in that manner. Comparing his wife to the woman whom he saw dressing in that manner is a very foolish thing to do. Most times, some spouses assume that when they compare their partners with other people, it is an effective way of pushing them to make necessary adjustments or shift to become like the person they are compared with.

Don't do that. It is not a wise thing to do at all.

In the same manner, it is an unwise thing to compare your husband to other men who did or bought something for their family as a way to compel him to do the same.

There are better ways to communicate your desires.

As a man, when you begin to buy her certain kind of clothes and compliment her every time she wears them, you have communicated.

Woman, appreciate your husband for the little you see him do. Shower him with appreciation and praise, and then make your request. He will wrest the moon to get that thing done or bring that thing home. Above all, pray for him always. He needs your prayers to get things done for the home and to keep the family running, he does not need pressure from comparison.

Sometimes, when you compare your partner to other people, it is a form of ingratitude. As much as you can, never allow yourself to say these words to your husband "What have you ever done for me?"

Those words will punch and deflate his morale.

For a woman, she receives comparison as a form of devaluation. It makes her lose her confidence and esteem.

Comparison is deadly. Because comparison can tamper with your spouse's esteem, it also can kill the bliss in your union.

CHAPTER THIRTEEN

MANAGING THIRD PARTIES

Marriage is a good thing that is designed for two people. A marriage does not happen except there are two people, not three.

One of the things that causes division in the home is third party. It is one of the things that has a quick effect in causing division in the home.

Before two people came together to get married, they were a product of a family. During this early stage of their life, they were at a stage of dependency. In the earliest stage, decisions were made for them. As they grow in this stage, they make decisions for themselves but these decisions were subject to the overarching principles that guided the family they belonged to and the home they lived. While still in this stage, the family they belonged to looked out for them on the kind of company they kept and the influence it had on them. And to some extent, there were shared concerns about how they used their time and restrictions on how much time they spent out.

Later, they exited that stage into independence. As independent adults, they made whole decisions for themselves. In this stage, they select their companies and choose their associations. To a large, restrictions are removed. Hence, the reason why it is called independence.

In marriage, two independent adults come together to submit their independence to each other thereby making them dependent on each other. Hence, they become interdependent.

Neither of the spouses is dependent on anybody other than their partner.

The family's control and parental influence ended in the dependent stage. Friend's company ended in the independent stage. Hence, a spouse is both a parent and a friend to his or her partner.

Listen, I am not saying that because you're now married, you should completely cut ties with your family and friends.

What I am saying is simple. Nobody should have your ears (attention) more than your partner. No one should occupy a space in your heart (affection) more than your partner. No one should have more of your time (quality time) than your partner. You cannot give to anyone more than you give to your partner.

Most times, third parties find access to your home when you go to them to seek advice. Most third parties are advisors who find their way into a couple's lives because the spouses are in disagreements, disgruntled, or suspicious of one another.

Generally, third parties should be avoided but, in the event, that you have to invite one because of a disagreement or misunderstanding that warrants it, ensure the third party whose counsel you seek is such that stems from the word of God. Their wisdom must be tested because it is so important that they cannot afford to take sides and level blame.

Secondly, it is important also that, when third parties have to be invited, the decision should be made by the couple. The man and the woman must agree to see a neutral person and talk about their disagreement with the person. This usually occurs when both parties are asserting their position or when there's a prolonged insistence on being right by both of them.

This is how to carefully select a third party.

If one partner decides to seek counsel from a third party without the knowledge, cooperation, or approval of the spouse, that will be a disaster waiting to happen. This is because the counsel that comes under such circumstances is likely going to be biased and full of prejudice. It usually brings about division. Do not open the third parties and allow yourself to discuss your marital issues with your colleague at work. Don't go to your mother or any of your family members and discuss your partner's inadequacies. These people love you but they don't live in your house, they will always see things the way you want them to see - your way, and for this reason, they will side with you.

You have a responsibility to cherish and honor your partner. Your partner is the first and topmost priority. No spouse wants to be second to his or her partner. This is what you would liken to God's command when He said "You shall not have other gods outside of me." God is a jealous God. Because we have the nature of God, we are jealous beings too. You build a safe relationship with your spouse when you don't cause them to feel unnecessarily jealous. You have to learn to be plain and open to your spouse. Avoid making your spouse jealous. Don't keep secrets. Jealousy creates bitterness and resentment.

Another area where the third-party idea is welcomed is when the couple finds another couple whose marriage they want to model theirs after. They can agree to both watch the couple from a distance and to have the couple talk with them as often as possible. Usually, this is to the end that their union will become better as what they get from the third party is wisdom for growth and bonding.

When I got married, I used to apologize to my friends every time because I couldn't meet up creating time to spend with them.

Gradually, I discovered that I won't be able to have time for them because my priorities have shifted. Slowly, they saw me pulled away. Thankfully, they understood.

As you grow, you will discover that you no longer delight in keeping company out there. Your delight will be in how much time you spend with your spouse.

CHAPTER FOURTEEN

SECRETS

This is one thing that will save you from making explanations that are not needed. You may not have ill intentions but when you start keeping secrets from your partner, you're gravitating towards giving room for distrust. When you make a slight mistake, you will speak so much "I can explain" and "It's not what you think." The simplest way to avoid these things is not to keep secrets from your partner.

Don't always assume you can handle everything. If your ex in your past relationships starts calling you or sending you messages, let your partner know about it. That way, the day your partner stumbles on a message from your ex in your brief absence, it won't make a difference. Better still, the day your partner bumps into your ex, anything your ex says to your partner won't make a difference.

You must realize that the forces that cause your marriage to fail are many out there. They are intentional about causing your marriage to fail and they are powerful more than you can handle on your own. It is the mystery power in unity that is stronger than all of them. This is why you cannot allow little secrets to cause division in your union.

If anything is troubling you, tell your spouse. You can surmount any challenge with the backing of your spouse. It is not your spouse that brings some special power that guarantees the victory, it is your union with your spouse that generates a mysterious power. Learn to pray, plan, and work together with your spouse. You cover more ground when you embark on a mission with your spouse. The Bible says that one can chase a thousand but when they come together in union, they create a rippling effect, they chase ten thousand.

The Bible says in Mark 3:25 "A house that is divided against itself cannot stand."

CHAPTER FIFTEEN

WRONG EXPECTATIONS

Marriage is anchored on love but there are aspects of it that are transactional.

How? You may want to ask.

Marriage is fifty-fifty, remember. One of these fifties is love (sacrificial) and the other fifty is transactional.

Marriage happens when there's an agreement between two adults in front of witnesses. The agreement and the presence of witnesses make the whole process transactional. The other side of marriage does not require agreement and it does not also require witnesses. It is the love aspect, and you know that love is sacrifice. It is incorrect to make a sacrifice for your spouse and expect the same to be done to you in return.

Not everything in marriage is transactional.

There's a quote by Mohit Hussein I want you to see. It says "Wrong expectations in a relationship lead to unnecessary disappointments."

Wrong expectations are the other side of the coin of comparisons. Listen to me, always remind yourself that the reason why you are married to your spouse is because of love. The reason why you are still together with your partner is because you're assured of love. Hence, anything you do in that marriage should be justified by love.

Lots of couples are sunk neck-deep in an unending quarrel because of expectations. The man says I bought you your favorite this and that during your last birthday but all you bought for me was just this. The woman says I have done this and that for you but just this thing I ask of you, you cannot do for me.

When you make your marriage about transactions, there will be so much manipulation. Let me remind you that love is selfless.

A transactional relationship between you and your spouse will make you both selfish because transactions are about motives - profits. It is not good to be married and be focused on what you can get only in the marriage.

If you're in your marriage for love, you will be focused on giving. Sacrifice is evident only in giving not receiving.

Let me categorically say this. It is witchcraft to do something for your spouse with the intent of getting the same or something similar done to you in return. In fact, it is occultic.

Sometimes, when I look at some ideas Christians have of Christianity, all I see is transaction. For example, "If I do this for God, God should do this for me in return." No, it shouldn't be so. Christianity is the fountain from where our idea about marriage flows because it is a marriage relationship between Jesus Christ and his us (His brides).

When you do something for God, is it because you want something in return or you out of love? Listen, God rewards. Just that, you don't determine the reward you should expect because a reward is simply a reward and not a paycheck. Your relationship with God is not contractual.

I have said all these to point out something to you. You will be destroying your marriage if you make it contractual. If you do your husband's laundry, it means you're entitled to $100. Isn't that ridiculous? Allow him to tell you thank you and reward you in the way he deems fit. In fact, the reward is not always instant. This is why you must learn to do things for your spouse out of a pure heart. Let your motive be sponsored by the love you have.

When you do something for your spouse, courtesy demands of him or her to say 'thank you.' Do not have expectations beyond a 'thank you.' Allow them to think of ways to reciprocate the gesture. If they don't reciprocate, it's still fine. After all, you didn't expect any reciprocation.

Your job in that marriage is to create a transformational relationship. As a man, you must become a transformational leader in your home. You're not a head to dish instructions only, everything must be channeled to the end that your spouse's life is becoming better by the day because of you. It is not different for the woman. Your husband must be able to count his blessings and place you in the top ranks. He should be able to say he has been able to do this and achieve that because he has you in his life.

CONCLUSION

Having a healthy marriage is not as simple as just wishing it into existence. It is a lifelong commitment to give a part of you into building a life and a home with your spouse.

It takes hard work and dedication by the partners involved, and a whole lot of God's grace. But your marriage doesn't have to be a chore; it can be a blast too!

With everything you have read in this book, I am persuaded that you gleaned on something that will make your marriage happy, healthy, and whole.

So, let's do a quick recap of each of the chapters in the book.

References

Mary DanPaul Fredericks, *When You are Ready*, Kaduna-Nigeria: Emergence Publishers, 2021.

Mercy Arinze Ezeugo, *The 50% Marriage Myths*. Kaduna-Nigeria: Emergence Publishers, 2021.

Dan Paul Fredericks, *When You are Married*, Kaduna-Nigeria: Emergence Publishers, 2021.

Deborah Tannen, "The Truth About How Much Women Talk – and Whether Men Listen," in *Time*. Accessed from https://www.google.com/amp/s/time.com/4837536/do-women-really-talk-more/%3famp=true 17th September, 2023.

Amy Roeder "Do Women Talk More Than Men?" in Harvard T. Chan, *School of Public Health* Accessed from https://www.hsph.harvard.edu/news/features/do-women-talk-more-than-men/ 17th September, 2023.

Sylvia Smith "5 Ways Lack of Compliments Ruin Your Marriage" in *Marriage.com* Accessed from https://www.marriage.com/advice/relationship/lack-of-appreciation/

Genesis 1:28

Proverbs 14:3 The Holy Bible

Proverbs 14:8 The Holy Bible

Proverbs 14:1 The Holy Bible

Proverbs 15:1 The Holy Bible

Proverbs 21:9 The Holy Bible

Deuteronomy 32:30 The Holy Bible

Isaiah 1:18, The Holy Bible

Proverbs 16:24 The Holy Bible

Matthew 18:22 The Holy Bible

Mark 3:25 The Holy Bible

Galatians 6:1 The Holy Bible